THE PSYCHOLOGY OF
MONEY

A Kid-Friendly Guide to Understand Money, Smart Choices, and Happiness!

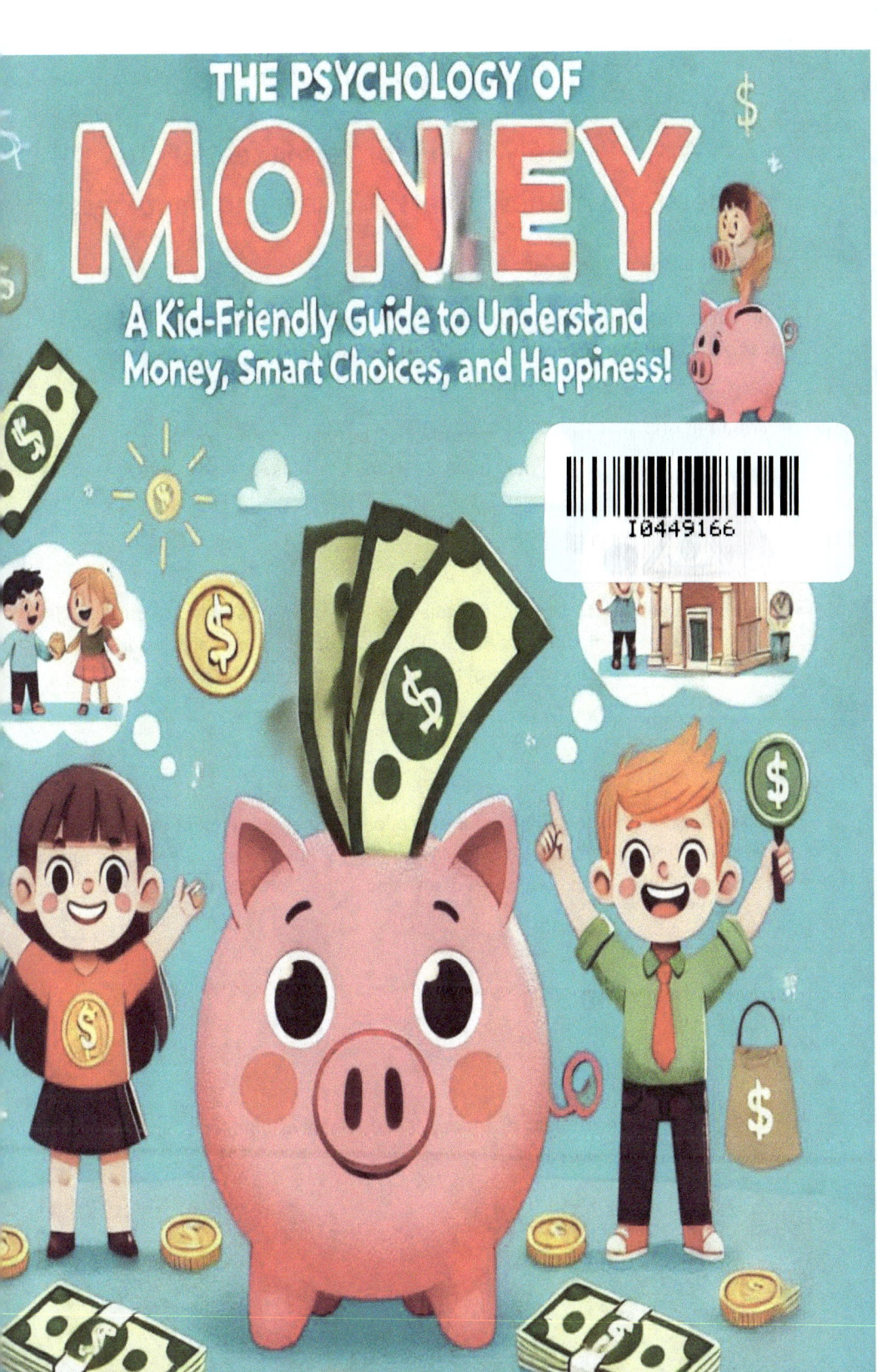

The Psychology of Money:

A Kid-Friendly Guide for young readers to understand money, smart choices, and happiness!

ISBN: 978-1-300-80927-2

Author: Benson G. Wilson

Book Title: The Psychology of Money: A Kid-Friendly Guide for young readers to understand money, smart choices, and happiness!

CONTENTS

No one is "crazy" about how they handle money. Everyone makes choices based on their own life, values, and what feels right to them. What might seem silly to one person could make perfect sense to someone else. We're all different, so we use money in different ways!

THREE SIMPLE STEPS TO FOLLOW

❖ *Understand Choices Are Personal:* Everyone makes their own choices about money based on what they think is important.

❖ *Respect Differences:* What you like might be different from what others like. One person might spend on toys; another might save for a trip.

❖ *Know That Beliefs Guide Choices:* People spend and save based on what they believe is right for them, even if it seems unusual to others.

EXAMPLE

If someone buys a fancy car, it might seem strange to you. But to them, it's something they really love and want to spend money on. And that's okay!

LESSON BREAKDOWN TO FOLLOW

- Choices are personal and based on what feels right.
- Respect that others may choose differently even if it's not what you would do.
- People spend based on beliefs and values that feel important to them.

Here's a picture of two kids, one putting money in a piggy bank and the other spending it on a toy. This shows that both options are fine.

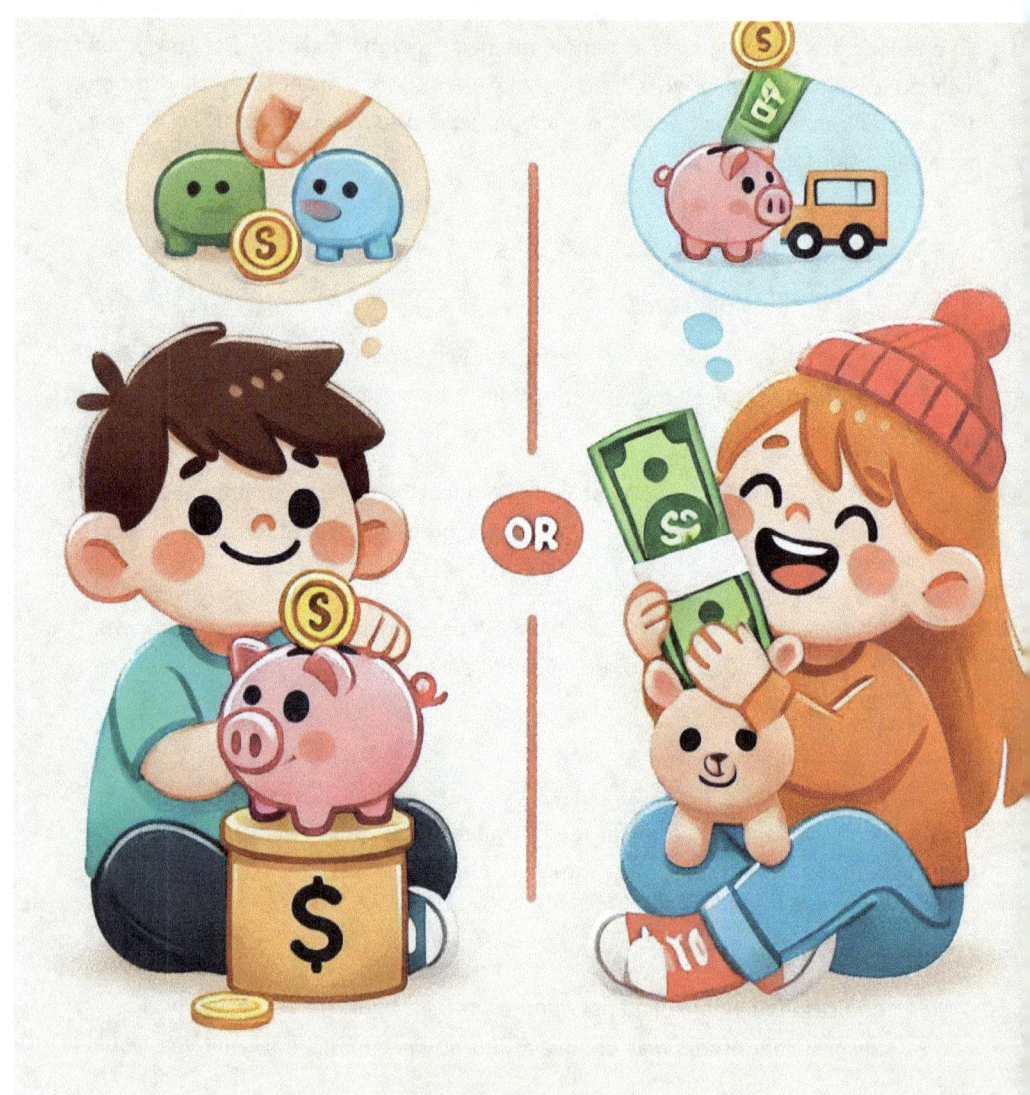

CHAPTER 2
LUCK & RISK

In life, luck and risk both play a big part! Sometimes, things turn out great just because of good luck, and other times things don't go well even if we try hard. This chapter explains that not everything is about effort. Sometimes, being in the right place at the right time or just a bit of luck makes a big difference.

THREE SIMPLE STEPS TO FOLLOW

❖ *Understand Luck's Role:* Realize that sometimes people succeed because they're lucky, not just because they worked hard.

❖ *Remember Risk:* Even with effort, things don't always go as planned. This is because there's always a little risk involved.

❖ *Focus on Effort, But Know Luck Helps:* Keep trying your best, but know that both luck and risk play a role in how things turn out.

EXAMPLE

If two friends play the same game, one might win just because they got a lucky start even though they both tried hard.

LESSON BREAKDOWN TO FOLLOW

- Luck sometimes helps people succeed even if others work just as hard.
- Risk means things don't always turn out the way we hope.
- Doing your best is great, but luck and risk are always there too.

Here's the illustration showing two children playing a game, with one child winning due to a lucky spin, demonstrating the role of luck.

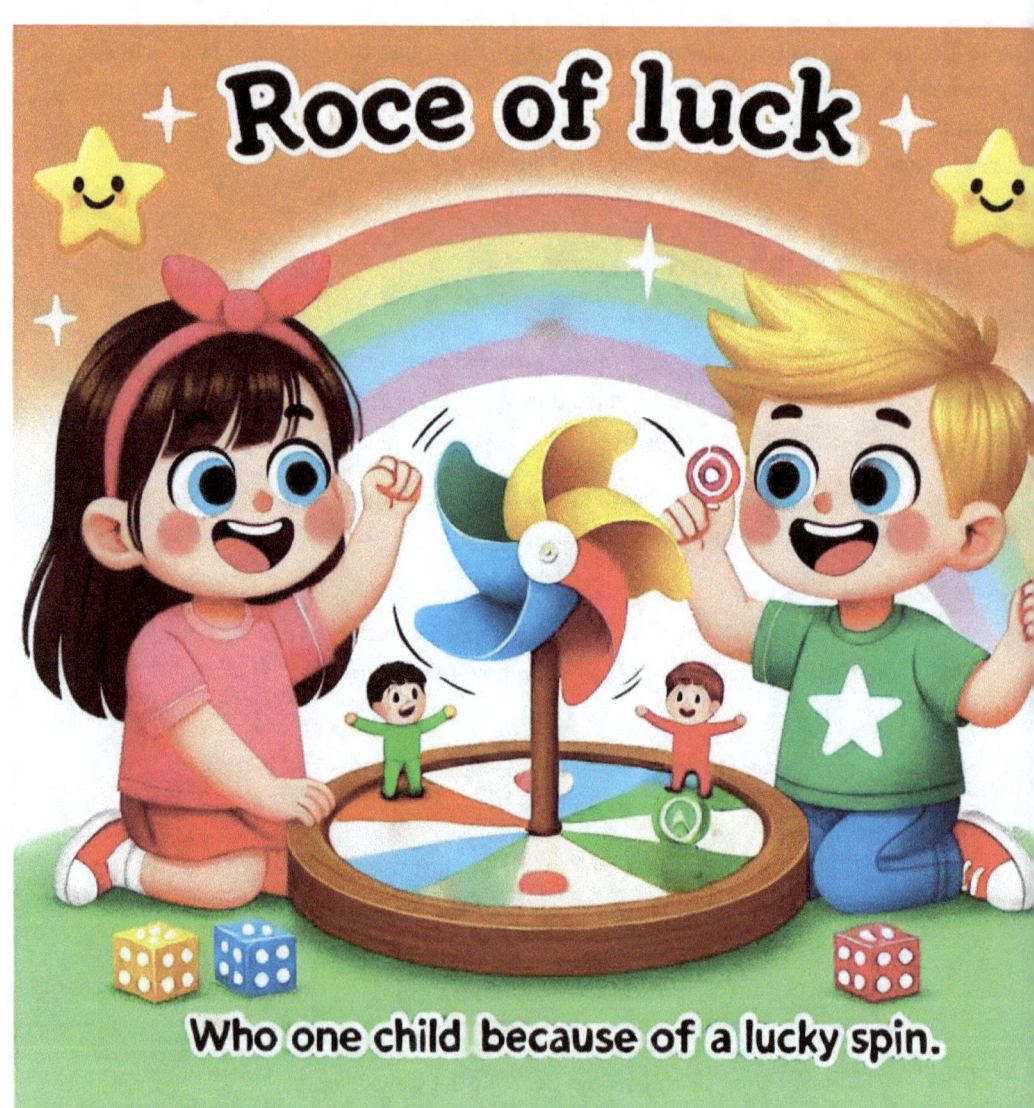

Roce of luck

Who one child because of a lucky spin.

CHAPTER 3
NEVER ENOUGH

This chapter explains that many people always want more money and things, but they don't know how much is "enough." Sometimes, even people with a lot of money keep wanting more. But if we don't know what "enough" is, we might never feel happy, no matter how much we have.

THREE SIMPLE STEPS TO FOLLOW

❖ *Think about What You Really Need:* Ask yourself what things make you happy and content, like having your favorite toys or time to play.

❖ *Learn to Be Happy with Enough:* Understand that always wanting more won't make you happier. Enjoy what you have!

❖ *Set Real Goals:* Decide what "enough" looks like for you, so you're not always chasing more.

EXAMPLE

If you get 10 candies, enjoy them! Don't keep asking for more if 10 already makes you happy.

LESSON BREAKDOWN TO FOLLOW
- Know what you need to feel happy.
- Enjoy what you have without always wanting more.
- Set a goal for what's "enough" so you can be happy with what you achieve.

This picture shows a child playing happily with their favorite toy, happy with having "enough."

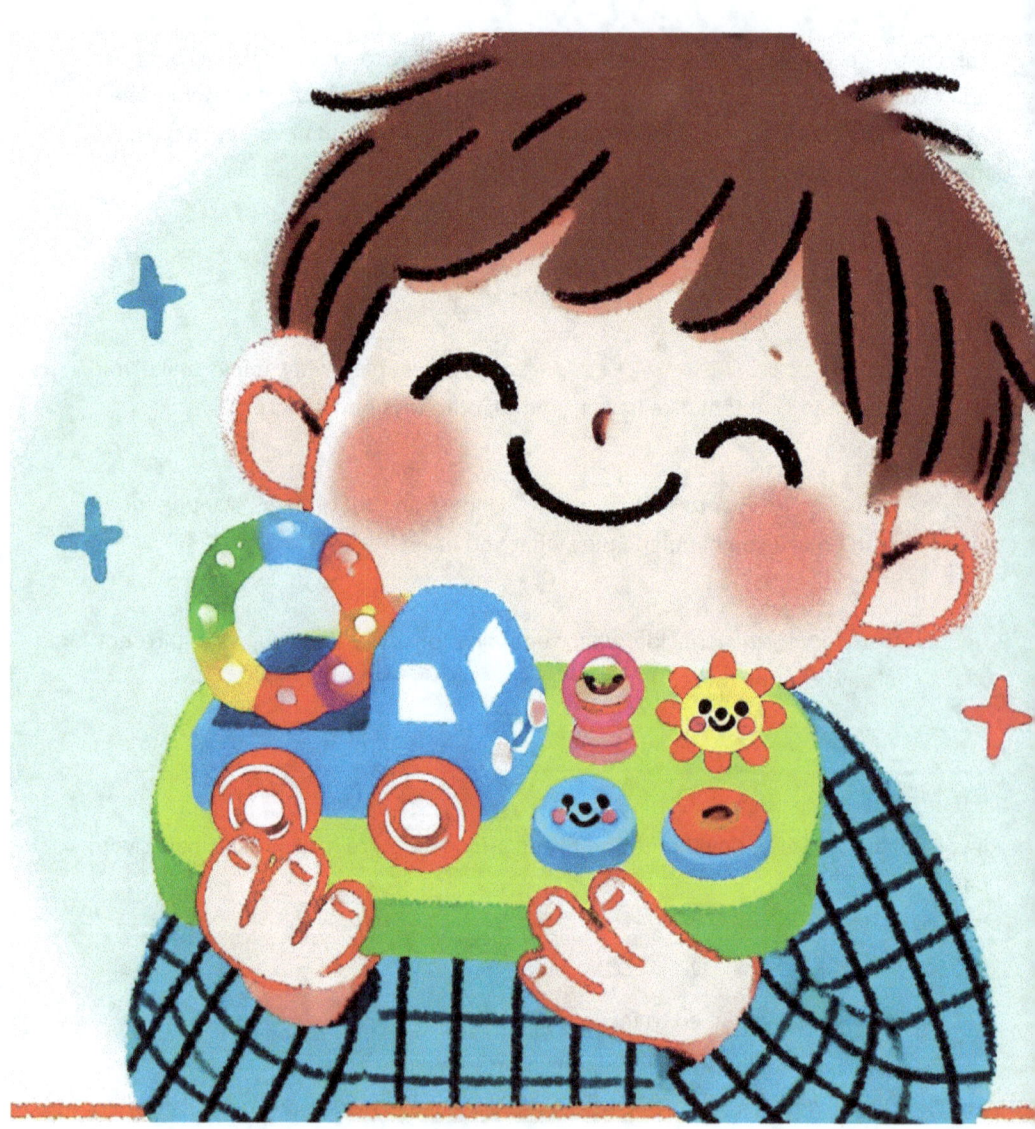

CHAPTER 4

THE MAGIC OF COMPOUNDING

Compounding is when small actions or savings grow bigger over time. Even if it doesn't seem like a lot at first, little things add up! For example, if you save a little bit every day, you'll have a lot after a year. Compounding helps us see that small, regular efforts can lead to big rewards later on.

THREE SIMPLE STEPS TO FOLLOW

❖ *Do a Little Each Day:* Small efforts, like saving a coin daily, can grow into something big over time.

❖ *Be Patient:* Compounding needs time to work, so keep going even if it seems slow.

❖ *Watch Your Progress:* Look back and see how far you've come to understand the power of small, steady steps.

EXAMPLE

If you read 5 pages every day, by the end of the year, you will have read a lot of books! Each day adds up, making you a better reader.

LESSON BREAKDOWN TO FOLLOW
- Start small and be consistent.
- Give it time to grow.
- See your improvement over time.

Here is the picture of a child who is happy to put a coin in a jar every day and watch it fill up over time.

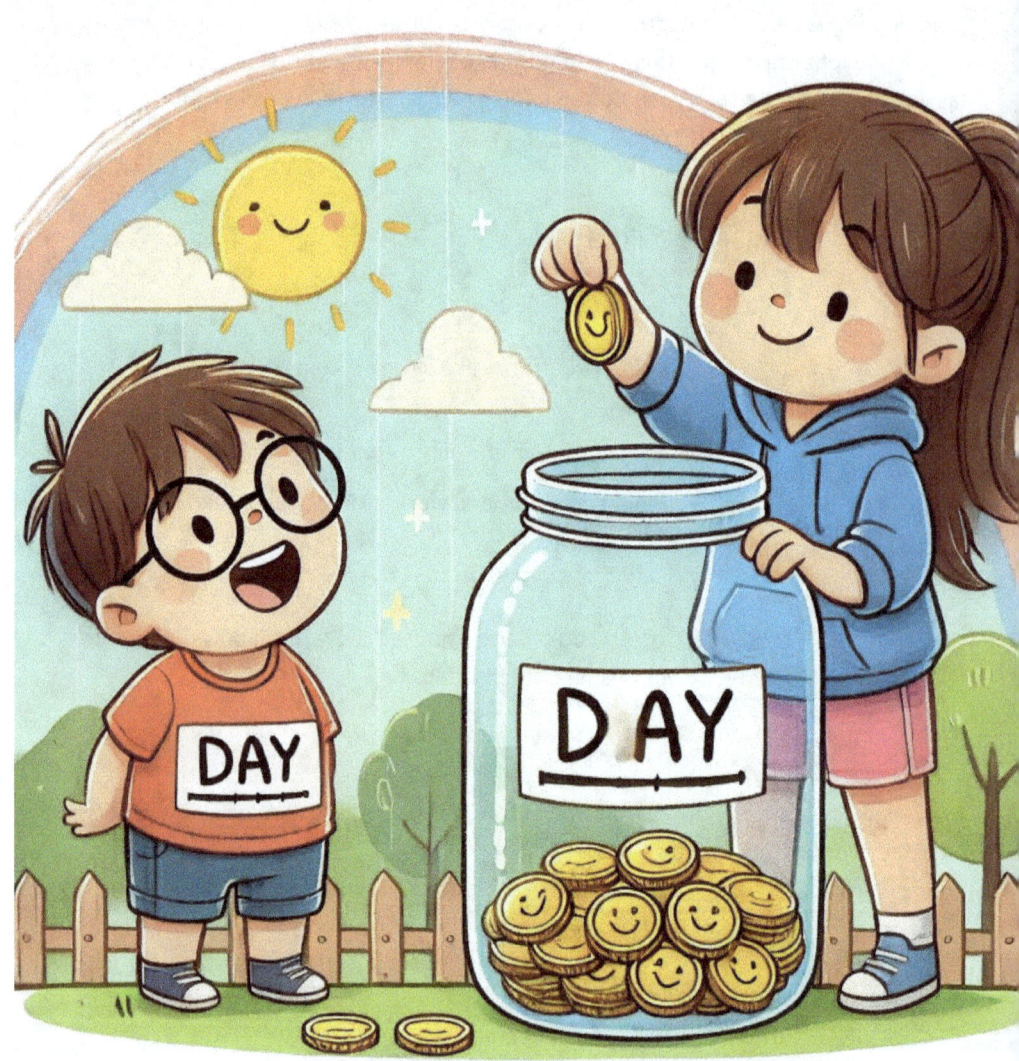

CHAPTER 5

GETTING WEALTHY VS. STAYING WEALTHY

Making money is one skill, but keeping that money is a different challenge. Many people know how to earn money, but saving it and making it last takes practice. This chapter shows that it's not only about earning money but also about making wise choices to keep it safe.

THREE SIMPLE STEPS TO FOLLOW

❖ *Learn to earn and Save:* Earning money is great, but saving is what keeps it safe for the future.

❖ *Avoid Big Mistakes:* Being careful with money helps you avoid losing it by making wise choices.

❖ *Think Long-Term:* To stay wealthy, focus on good habits that help you keep money safe over time.

EXAMPLE

If you earn money by doing chores, saving a part of it each time instead of spending all of it will help you keep it for something special.

LESSON BREAKDOWN TO FOLLOW

- Earning is only the start; saving helps keep money for the future.
- Make careful choices to avoid losing money quickly.
- Build long-term habits to keep your savings safe.

This picture of a child putting some of their pay into a piggy bank shows how important it is to both earn money and save it.

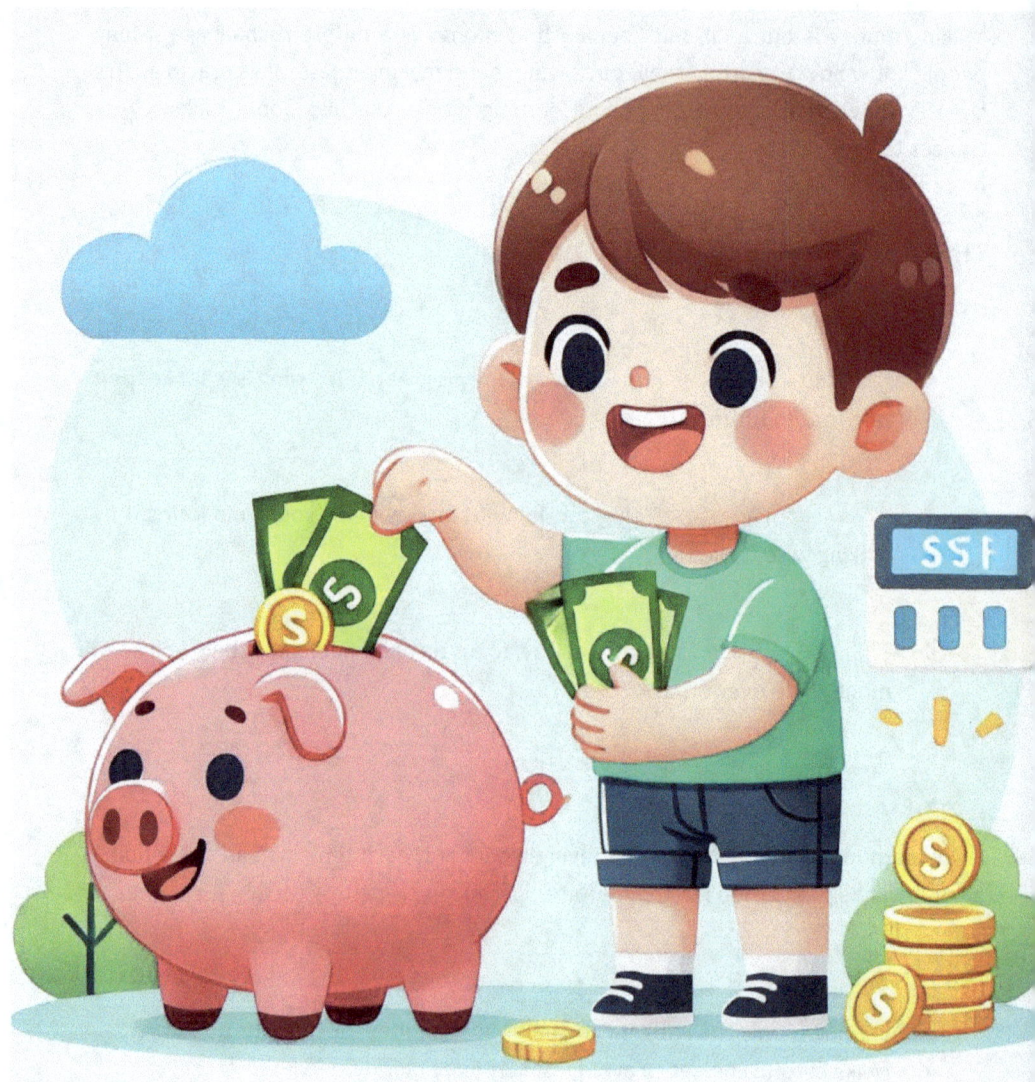

CHAPTER 6

TAILS, YOU WIN

In this chapter, the author explains that it's okay to make mistakes when trying to earn or save money. Even big companies like Amazon have made mistakes, but they didn't give up! Instead, they kept trying and eventually found success. The key is to keep going, even if things don't work out at first.

THREE SIMPLE STEPS TO FOLLOW

❖ *Learn from Mistakes:* Understand that it's okay to make mistakes. Mistakes help you learn and get better.

❖ *Keep Trying:* If something doesn't work out, don't give up. Keep trying different ways to succeed.

❖ *Focus on the Wins:* Even if you lose sometimes, keep looking for chances to win in the long run.

EXAMPLE

If you try a new game and lose a few times, don't get discouraged. With practice, you'll get better and start winning!

LESSON BREAKDOWN TO FOLLOW

- Mistakes are okay because they help you learn.
- Keep trying even if things don't go perfectly at first.
- Success can come after some losses, so keep looking for your next win.

This picture shows a child playing a game. They lose one round but keep happy and try again, which shows they are persistent.

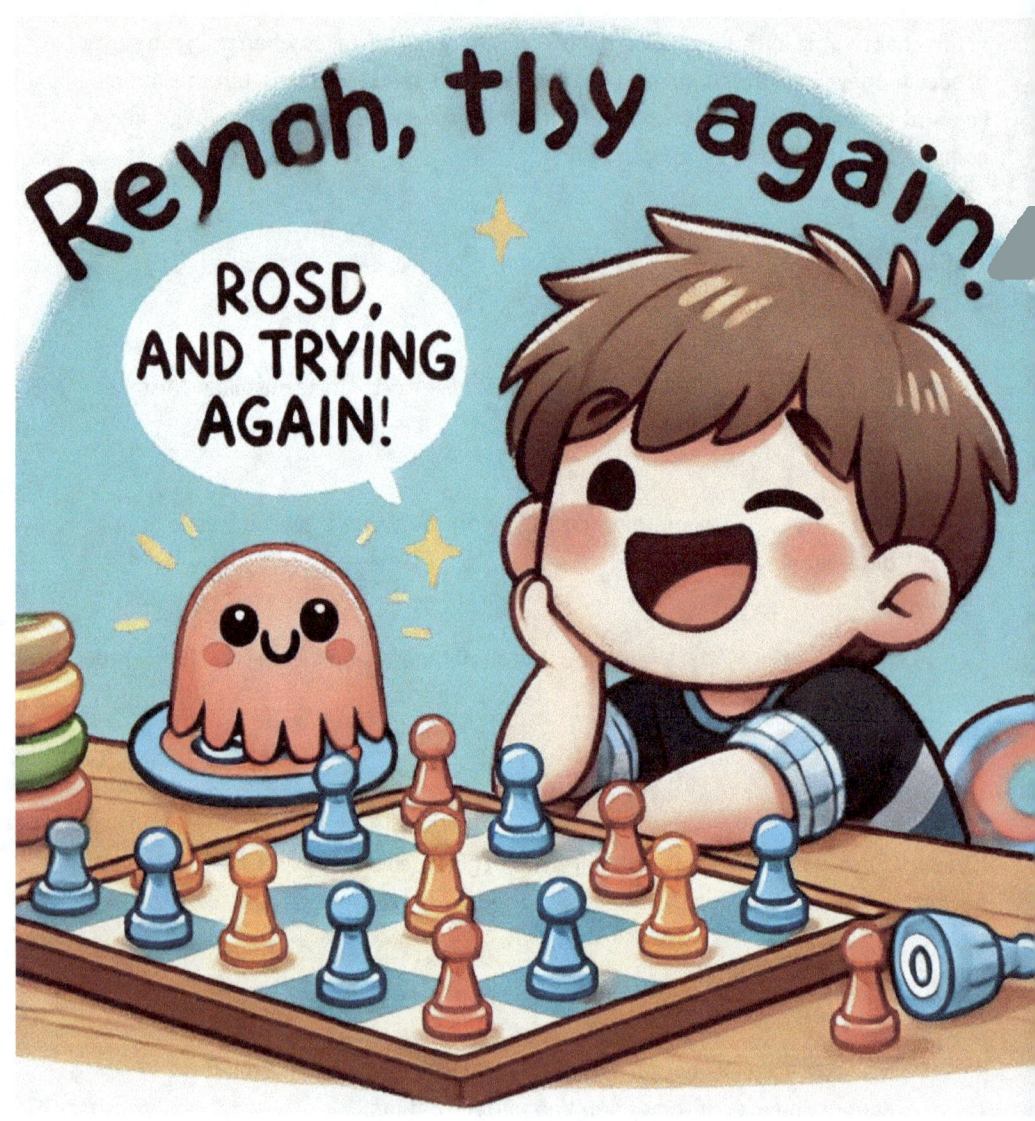

CHAPTER 7
FREEDOM

Money is helpful, but true wealth is having the freedom to use your time as you want! The author explains that having control over your time and feeling free is way more valuable than just having a lot of money. The best thing about money is that it can give you freedom to do the things you love.

THREE SIMPLE STEPS TO FOLLOW

❖ *Think About What Makes You Happy*: Money is good, but it's more important to have time to enjoy your life and do what makes you happy.

❖ *Use Money to Gain Freedom:* Use money to make choices that give you more freedom, like spending time with family or friends.

❖ *Remember, Money Isn't Everything:* Money helps, but happiness and freedom are even more valuable.

EXAMPLE

Imagine if you earned a lot of money but never had time to play with friends or do your favorite hobbies. Money is great, but having the time to enjoy it is even better!

LESSON BREAKDOWN TO FOLLOW

- Focus on what brings happiness and freedom.
- Use money wisely to make time for things you love.
- Money alone doesn't bring happiness; it's freedom that counts.

Here's the illustration showing a child enjoying free time in the park with friends, highlighting that freedom is as valuable as money.

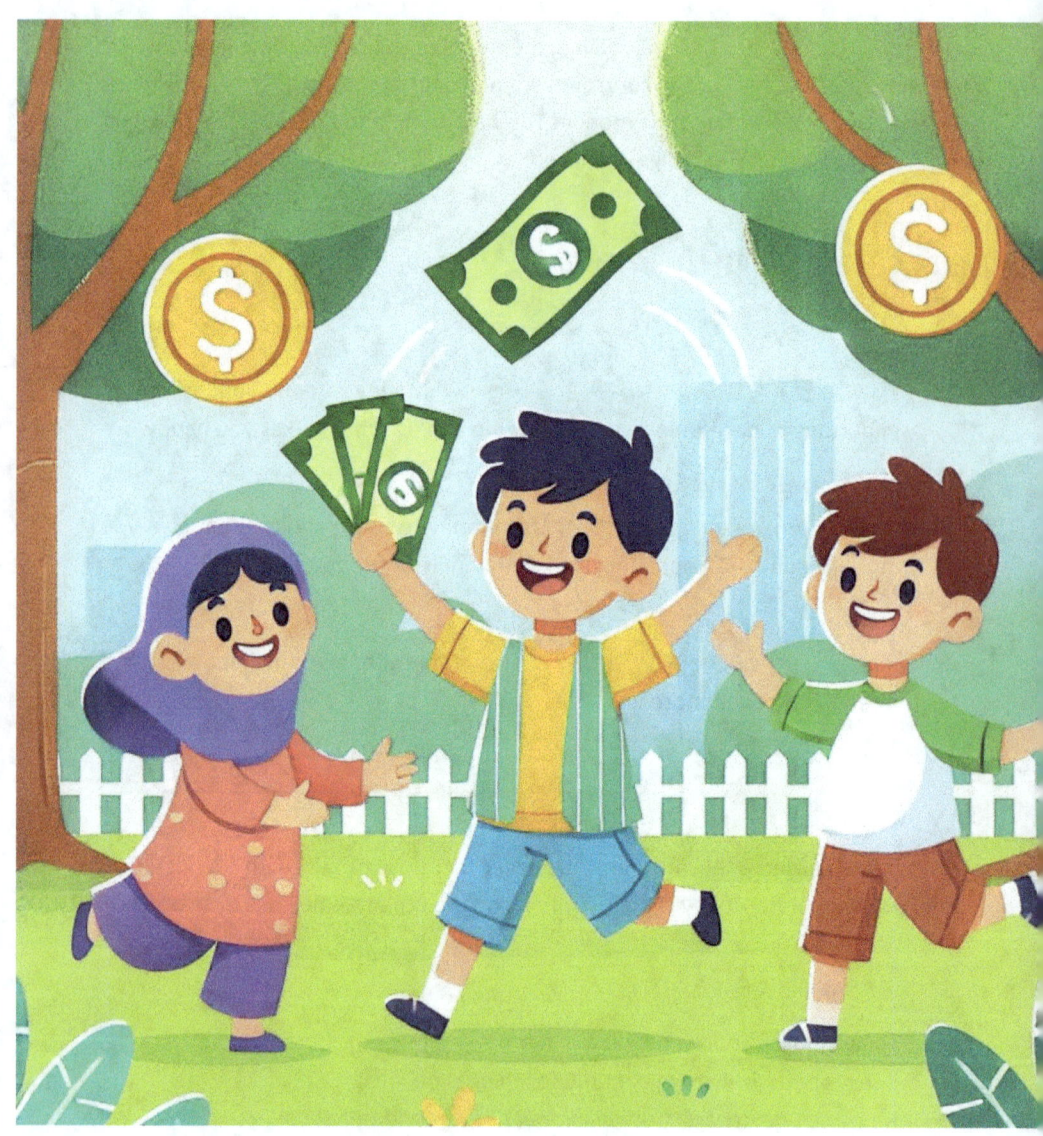

CHAPTER 8

THE CAR PARADOX

Some people think that showing off their fancy things will make others admire them. But often, it doesn't work that way! People don't really care about your cool stuff as much as you think. True respect and friendship come from who you are, not what you own.

THREE SIMPLE STEPS TO FOLLOW

- ❖ *Remember What Really Matters:* People like you for who you are, not for the things you own.

- ❖ *Be Kind, Not Flashy:* True friends care about you, not about your cool toys or clothes.

- ❖ *Spend Wisely:* Save money for things that make you happy, not just to impress others.

EXAMPLE

If you buy a really cool toy to impress your friends, they might think it's fun, but they'll like you because of your kindness and friendship, not just your toy.

LESSON BREAKDOWN TO FOLLOW

- People like you for being kind and friendly, not for what you have.
- True friendships come from who you are on the inside.
- Spend wisely on things that make you happy, not just to show off.

This picture shows a child playing a simple game with friends while being happy. It shows that friendships are more important than fancy things.

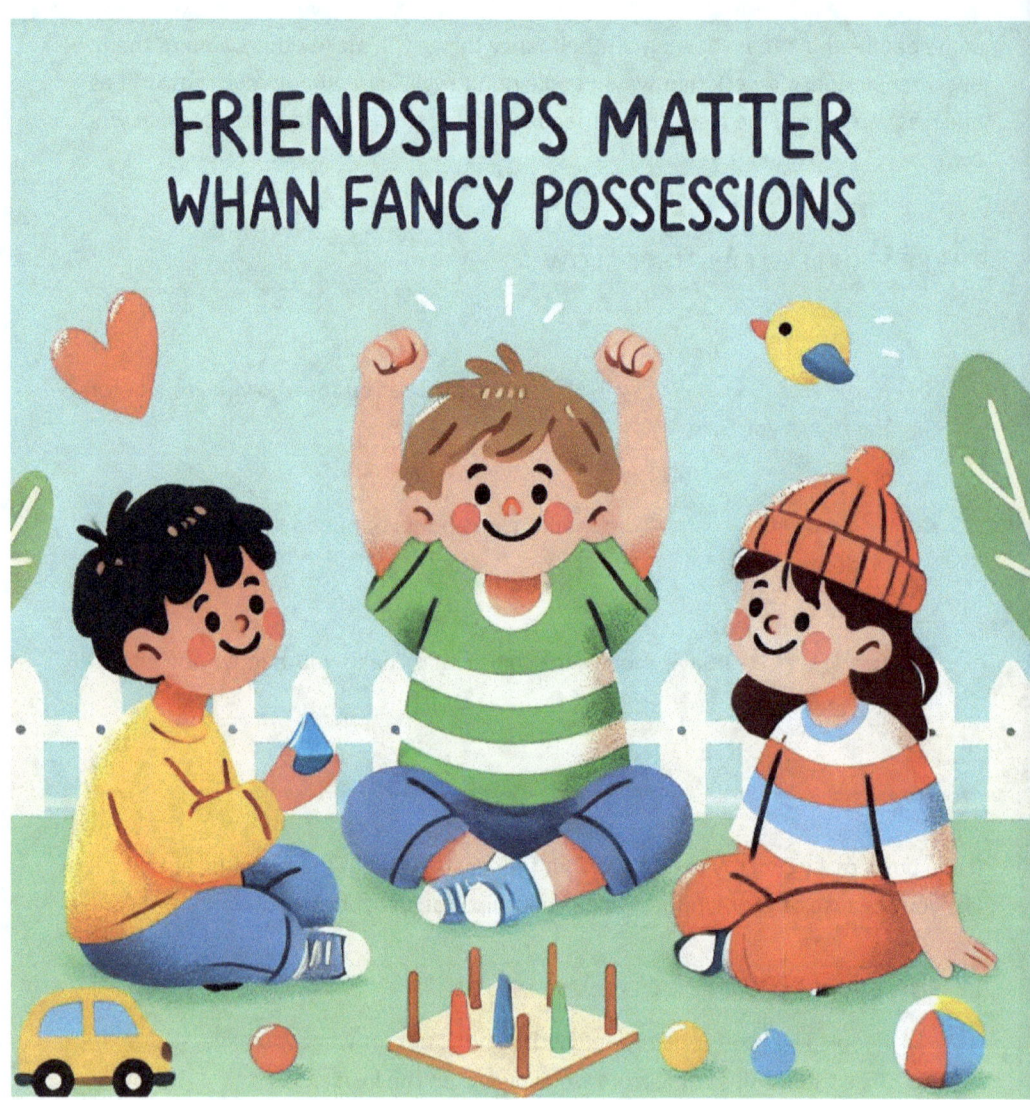

CHAPTER 9

Wealth isn't just about spending lots of money on fancy things. Some people think showing off expensive items makes them look rich, but actually, saving money and using it wisely is what makes someone truly wealthy. Real wealth means having money saved for the future, not just spending it all at once.

THREE SIMPLE STEPS TO FOLLOW

❖ *Understand True Wealth:* Wealth means having money saved, not just spending it to look rich.

❖ *Be Smart with Money:* Instead of buying fancy things, try to save for things that matter to you.

❖ *Remember, it's What You Don't See:* True wealth is often hidden in smart savings, not in flashy things.

EXAMPLE

If you save your allowance each week, you're building wealth. But if you spend it all on toys, you won't have anything saved for later.

LESSON BREAKDOWN TO FOLLOW

❖ Wealth is about saving, not just spending on fancy things.
❖ Think about what matters when you choose to spend or save money.
❖ Real wealth grows when you make wise choices with money.

Here's the illustration of a child happily putting money into a piggy bank while other children play with toys, showing that saving can lead to future wealth.

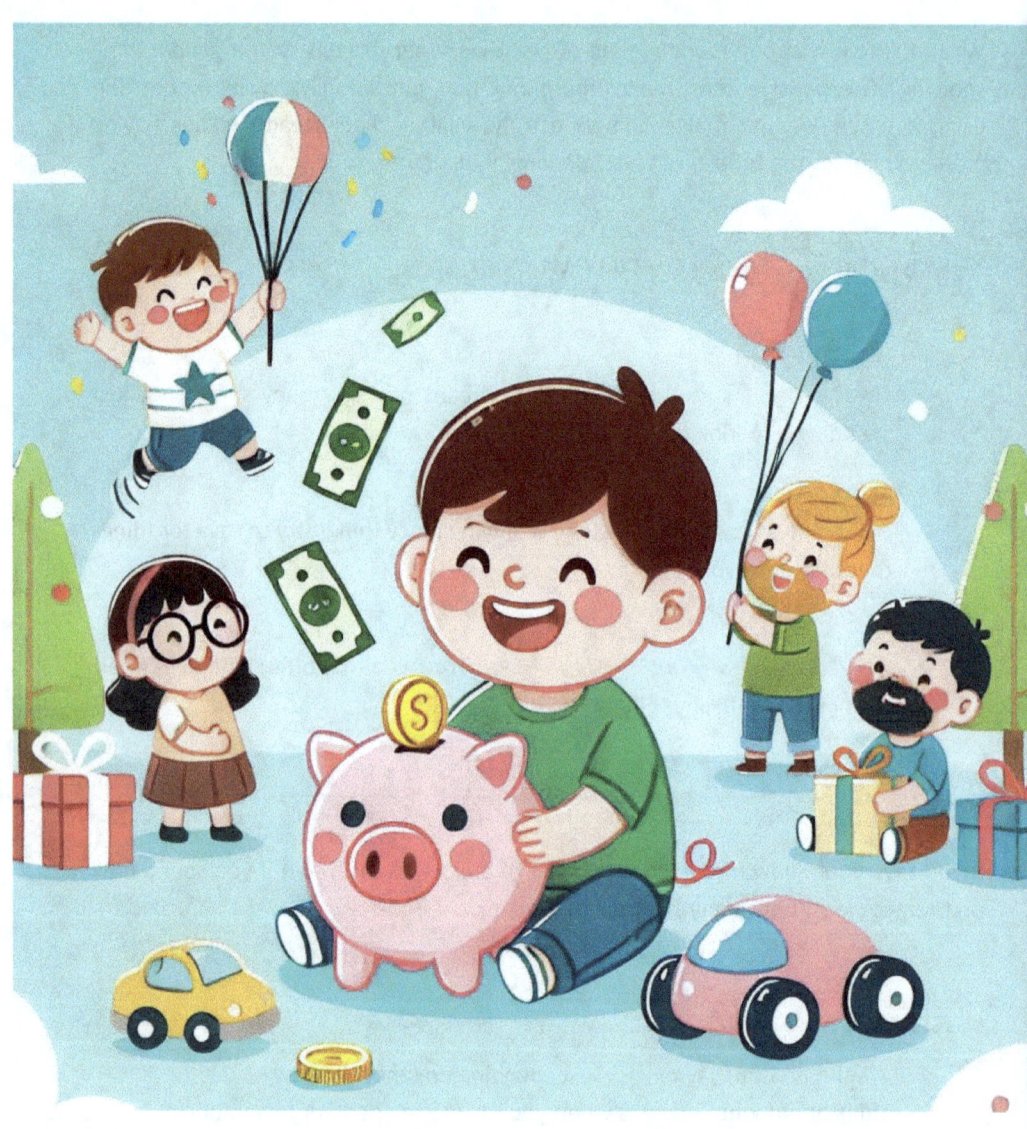

CHAPTER 10

SAVE MONEY

Saving money is really important because nothing in life is truly free. Even things that seem free have some kind of cost. The author explains that the value of something isn't always about the price tag. It's about how useful or important it is to you.

THREE SIMPLE STEPS TO FOLLOW

❖ *Understand Value:* Some things may seem free, but they often have hidden costs. Learn to look at the real value of things.

❖ *Think Before You Spend:* When you save money, you can buy things that are truly valuable to you.

❖ *Appreciate the Priceless Things:* Not everything valuable has a price tag, like friendship, family, and freedom.

EXAMPLE

Imagine you get a free toy from a friend, but now you need to spend time taking care of it. So, even though it was free, it still comes with a cost!

LESSON BREAKDOWN TO FOLLOW

- Nothing is completely free; there's always some kind of cost.
- Save money to buy things that are truly valuable to you.
- Remember that priceless things like freedom and friendships are the most valuable.

This drawing shows a child carefully putting coins into a piggy bank while thinking about a toy that has secret prices. It shows how important it is to save money and know what things are worth.

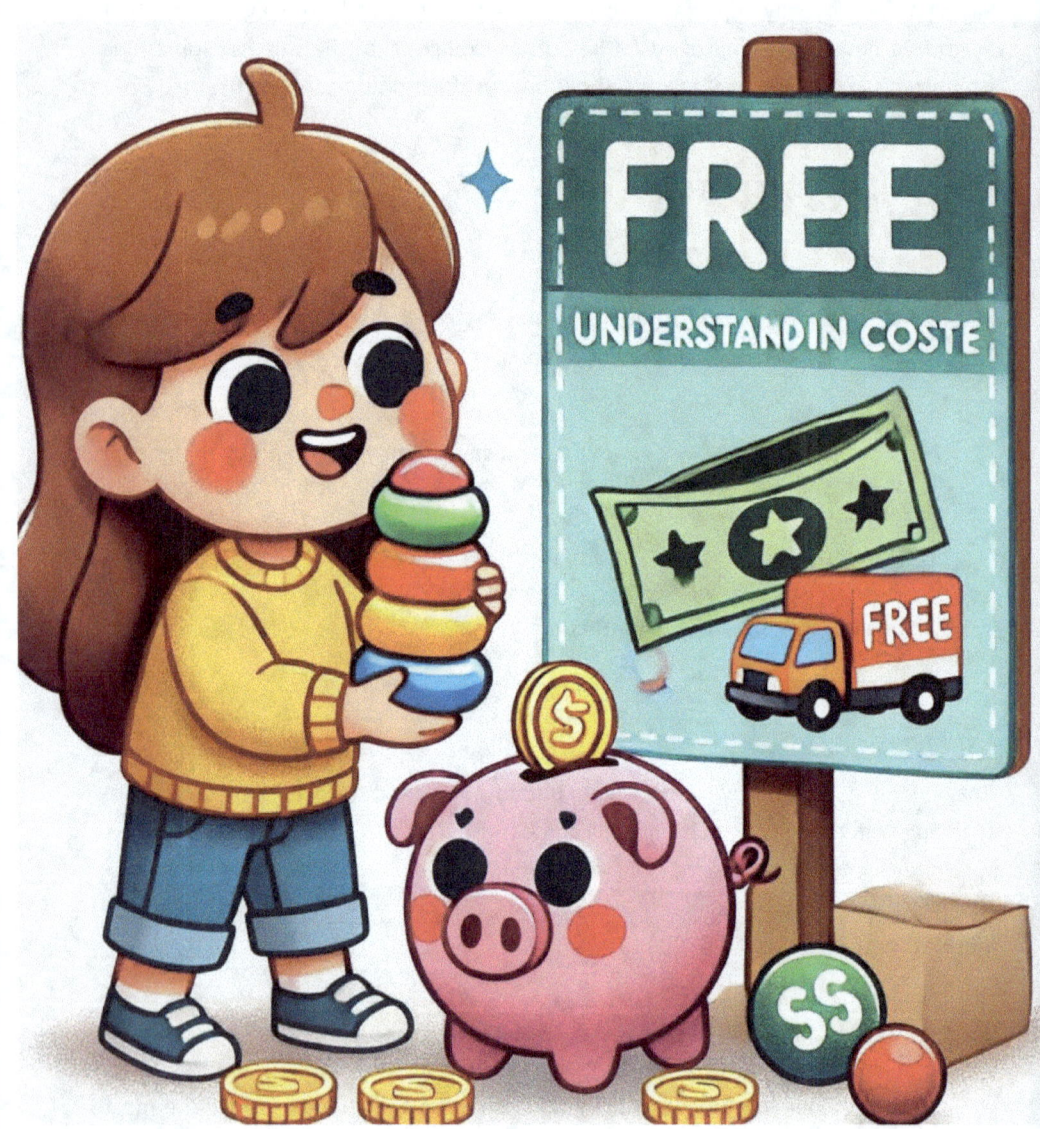

CHAPTER 11

REASONABLE VS. RATIONAL

Being reasonable means making choices that feel right and are sensible, even if they don't follow strict logic. Instead of always focusing on "perfect" decisions, it's often better to make choices that are good for you and others. Trying to be perfectly logical or "rational" might not always be helpful!

THREE SIMPLE STEPS TO FOLLOW

❖ *Think About What Feels Right:* It's okay to go with what feels sensible, even if it's not "perfect."

❖ *Balance Thinking and Feeling:* Sometimes, making a choice that feels fair or caring is better than just following strict rules.

❖ *Make Decisions That Help You and Others:* Being reasonable means choosing what's best overall, not just what's perfectly logical.

EXAMPLE

Imagine choosing between giving a friend half of your snack or keeping it all. Reasonable thinking might say, "I'll share because it's fair and makes my friend happy," rather than "keeping it is more logical for me."

LESSON BREAKDOWN FOR KIDS:

- Being reasonable means making kind, sensible choices, not always focusing on strict rules.
- Consider how a decision affects you and others.
- Being reasonable can be more helpful than always aiming for perfect logic.

There is a picture of a child sharing a snack with a friend to show that being reasonable and fair is sometimes more helpful than just using logic.

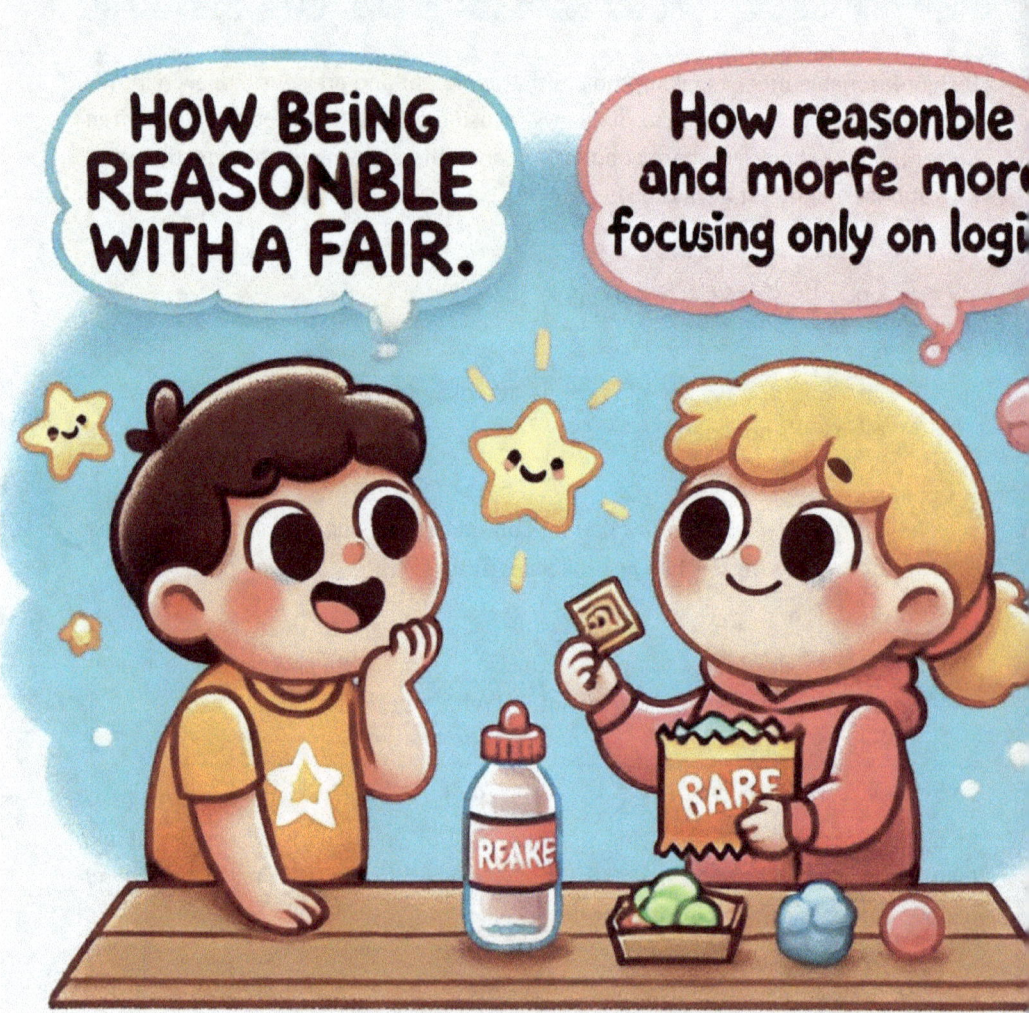

CHAPTER 12

EXPECT SURPRISES

Life is full of surprises! Sometimes things don't go exactly as planned, and that's okay. History is like a story of all the changes people have gone through. Even though it teaches us a lot, it doesn't tell us exactly what will happen in the future.

THREE SIMPLE STEPS TO FOLLOW

❖ *Learn from the Past:* History teaches us about changes, but it doesn't give all the answers for what's next.

❖ *Be Ready for Surprises:* Things don't always go as planned, so stay flexible and open to new things.

❖ *Keep a Positive Mindset:* Surprises can be fun and help us learn, so try to enjoy them!

EXAMPLE

Imagine planning a fun day at the park, but it starts to rain. You can still have a great day by playing indoor games or watching a movie instead.

LESSON BREAKDOWN TO FOLLOW

- Learn from what's happened before, but be open to new surprises.
- Stay flexible and creative when things don't go as planned.
- Enjoy surprises as a chance to learn and grow.

Here's the illustration of children happily adapting to a rainy day by playing indoor games, showing how fun it can be to stay flexible and enjoy surprises.

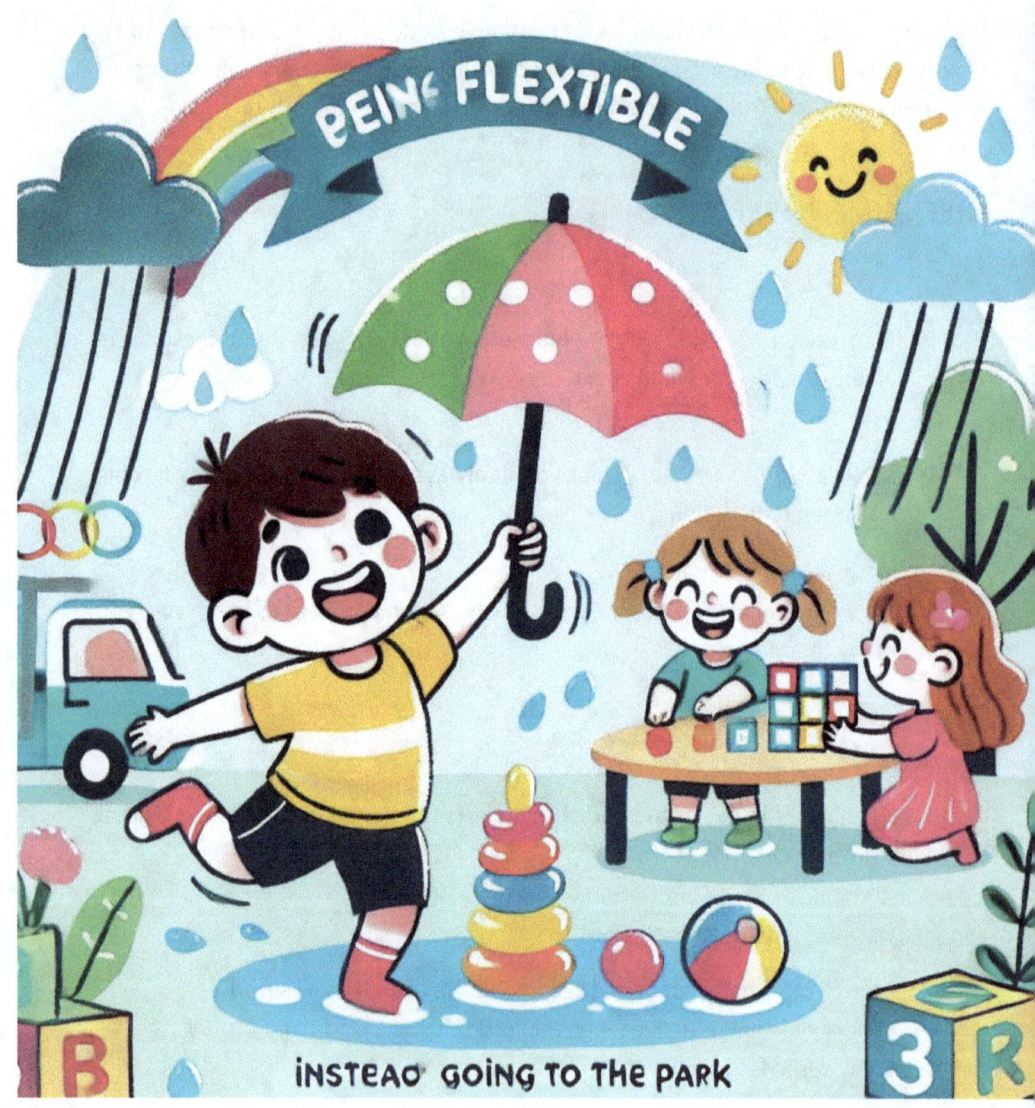

CHAPTER 13

MAKE ROOM FOR MISTAKES

When we make a plan, it's smart to leave space for things to go differently than expected. Sometimes, even the best plans don't work out perfectly, and that's okay! Being ready for little mistakes or changes can help us handle surprises better.

THREE SIMPLE STEPS TO FOLLOW

❖ *Expect Changes:* Understand that plans don't always go perfectly. It's okay to adjust!

❖ *Stay Calm if Things Change:* Don't worry if something unexpected happens. Think of new ways to make it work.

❖ *Learn from Mistakes:* Use any surprises or changes as a chance to learn and make even better plans next time.

EXAMPLE

Imagine planning to make a tall building out of blocks, but it keeps falling. You can learn to build it shorter and sturdier so it stays up!

LESSON BREAKDOWN TO FOLLOW

- Plans sometimes change, so be ready to adjust.
- Stay calm and find new ideas when things go differently.
- Use mistakes as learning moments to improve for next time.

This picture shows a child who tried to build a bigger tower out of blocks but failed and ended up making a shorter, stronger one instead. This shows that making mistakes and learning from them can lead to better results.

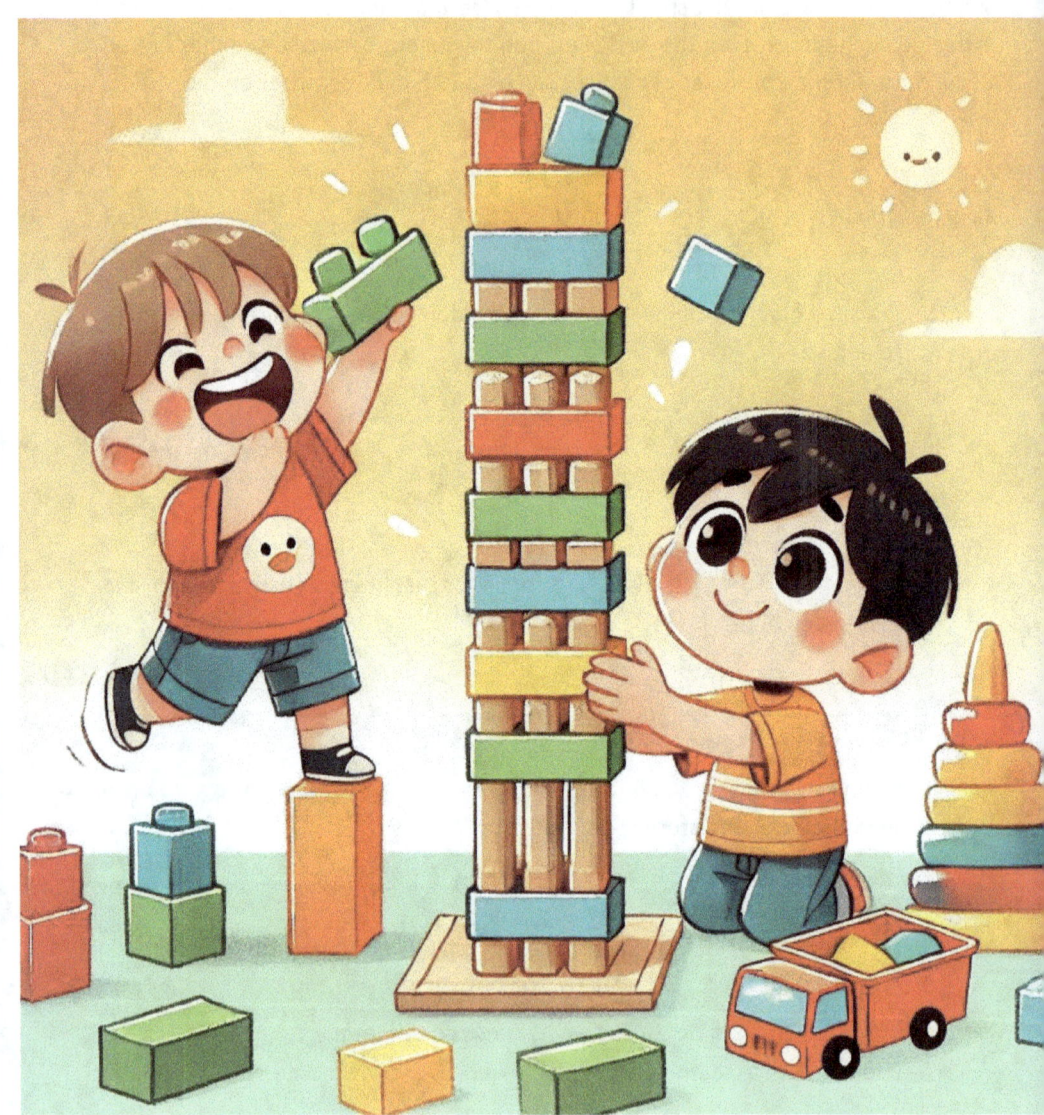

CHAPTER 14

YOU'LL CHANGE OVER TIME

When we make plans for the future, we often think we'll always want the same things. But as we grow, our goals and interests can change, and that's normal! It's okay if you don't want the same things you used to; being flexible with your plans is important.

THREE SIMPLE STEPS TO FOLLOW

❖ *Make Plans, But Be Open to Change:* It's great to have goals, but be ready to adjust as you grow.

❖ *Listen to Your New Interests:* If you start liking new things, it's okay to change your plans to match those.

❖ *Remember, Change Helps You Grow:* Changing your goals can help you learn more about yourself.

EXAMPLE

Imagine you dream of being a firefighter, but later you discover a love for painting. It's okay to switch your dream and make new goals that fit who you are now.

LESSON BREAKDOWN TO FOLLOW

- Plans may change as you grow—and that's perfectly okay!
- Adjust your goals if new interests make you happy.
- Changing goals is a way to learn about yourself and find what you truly enjoy.

Here's the illustration of a child holding a drawing of being a firefighter, then happily painting something new, showing how interests can change over time.

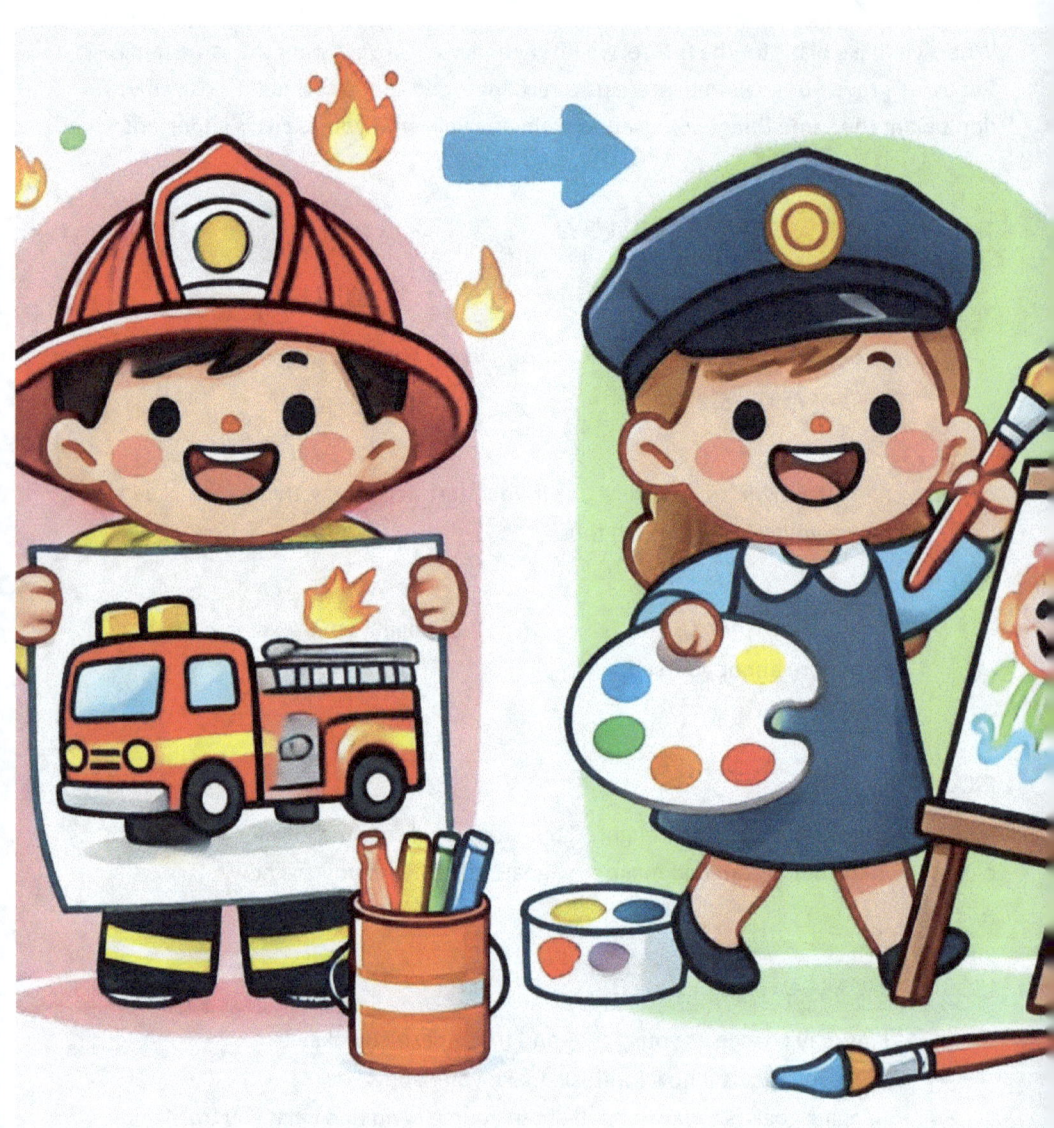

CHAPTER 15

NOTHING IS REALLY FREE

Sometimes things seem free, but there's usually a cost we don't see right away. The price of something isn't always just money; it can be time, effort, or other things we give up. Understanding that everything has a cost helps us make better choices.

THREE SIMPLE STEPS TO FOLLOW

❖ *Look beyond the Label:* Remember that even if something seems free, it might have a hidden cost.

❖ *Think About What You're Giving Up:* It could be your time, energy, or something else valuable.

❖ *Choose Wisely:* Make choices that are worth the cost, even if you don't see it right away.

EXAMPLE

Imagine a friend offers you a free snack but asks for half your lunch in return. The snack isn't really free you're giving up part of your lunch!

LESSON BREAKDOWN TO FOLLOW

- Understand that everything has a price, even if it doesn't look like it.
- Consider what you might give up when taking something that seems free.
- Make smart choices based on what you're really getting and giving up.

Here's the illustration showing a child being offered a "free" snack but understanding it takes trading part of their lunch, teaching that nothing is truly free.

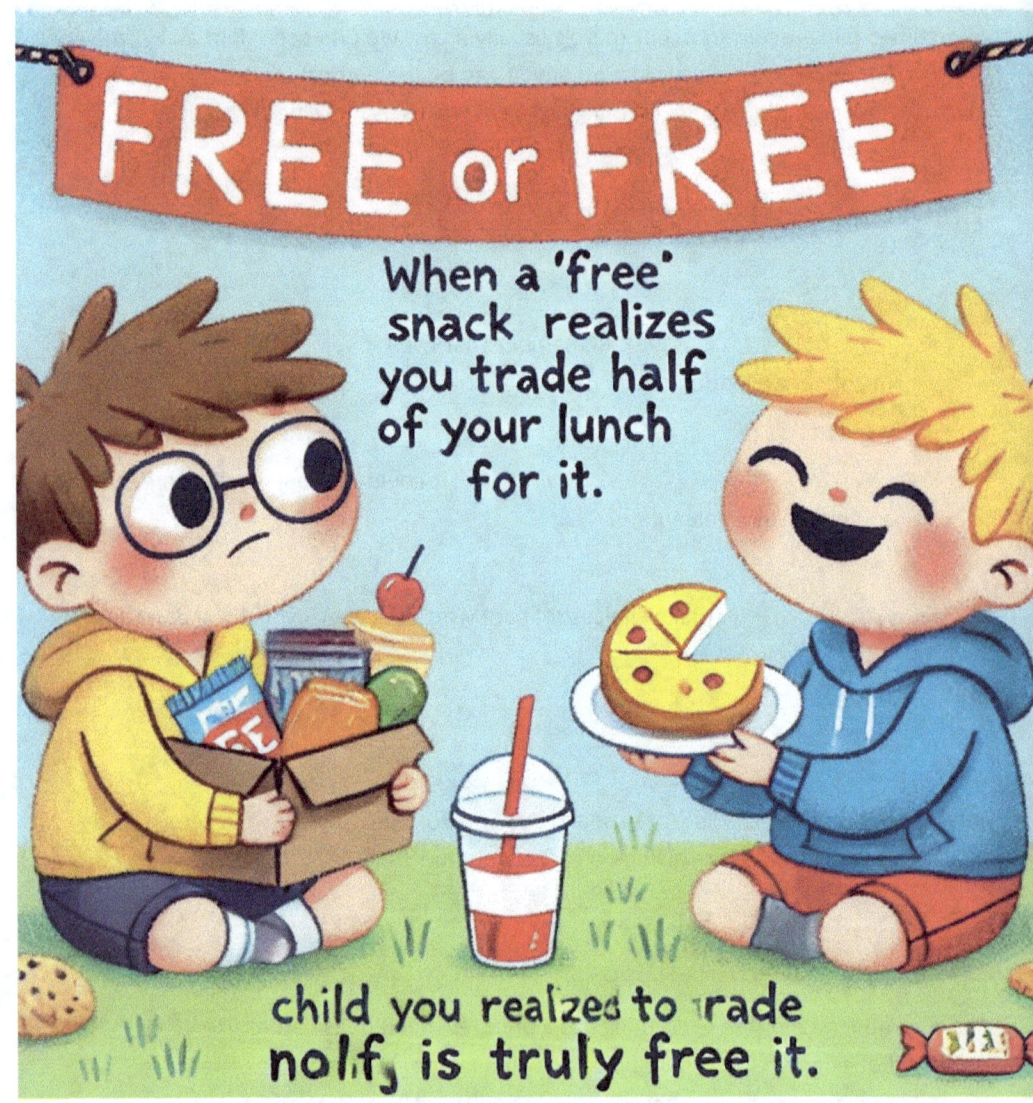

CHAPTER 16

YOU & ME - PLAYING DIFFERENT GAMES

Everyone has different goals and plans, so it's important not to copy what others do with money if they're aiming for different things. What works for someone else may not work for you because you might have different dreams and needs.

THREE SIMPLE STEPS TO FOLLOW

❖ *Remember Your Own Goals:* Think about what you want to achieve rather than what others are doing.

❖ *Ask Questions:* Before following someone else's choices, think about if it's right for you.

❖ *Make Choices That Match Your Path:* Stick with plans that help you reach your own dreams, not just because others are doing it.

EXAMPLE

If a friend spends all their money on toys, it might not be the best idea for you if you're saving up for a new bike. You both have different goals!

LESSON BREAKDOWN TO FOLLOW

- Understand that everyone has unique goals and needs.
- Make choices that match your own dreams, not just what others are doing.
- Think about your own "game" and plan for it.

This picture shows a child saving money for a bike in a piggy bank, while another child uses their money on toys. This shows that everyone has different goals.

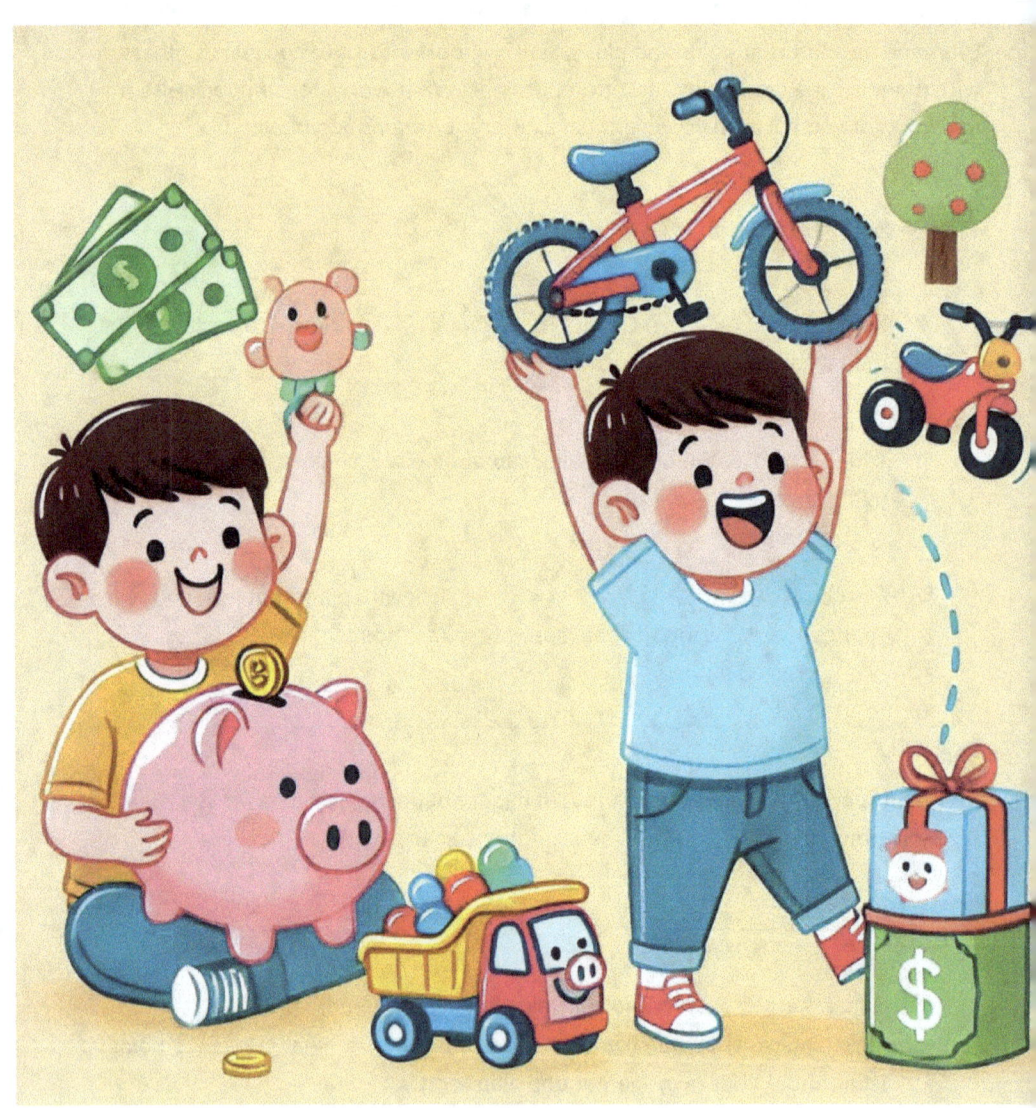

CHAPTER 17
THE PULL OF PESSIMISM

Sometimes, it feels safer to think things might go wrong. People often believe someone who says, "Be careful, this might not work!" more than someone who says, "It will be great!" But always expecting bad things can stop us from trying new ideas and learning.

THREE SIMPLE STEPS TO FOLLOWS

❖ *Listen, But Don't Let Fear Stop You:* It's okay to hear warnings, but don't let them scare you from trying.

❖ *Believe in Possibilities:* Give new ideas a chance, even if someone is worried it won't work.

❖ *Balance Optimism and Caution:* Be hopeful, but also careful. This helps you make smart choices without being too afraid.

EXAMPLE

Imagine a friend says, "That new game might be too hard, so don't try it." Another friend says, "You'll do great, give it a go!" It's okay to be careful, but you'll only know how fun it is if you try.

LESSON BREAKDOWN TO FOLLOW

- Understand the difference between warnings and encouragement.
- Don't let worry hold you back from new experiences.
- Balance hope and caution to make the best decisions.

Here's the illustration showing one child looking worried and saying, "That slide might be too tall," while another friend encourages, "Let's give it a try, it could be fun!" This captures the balance between caution and optimism.

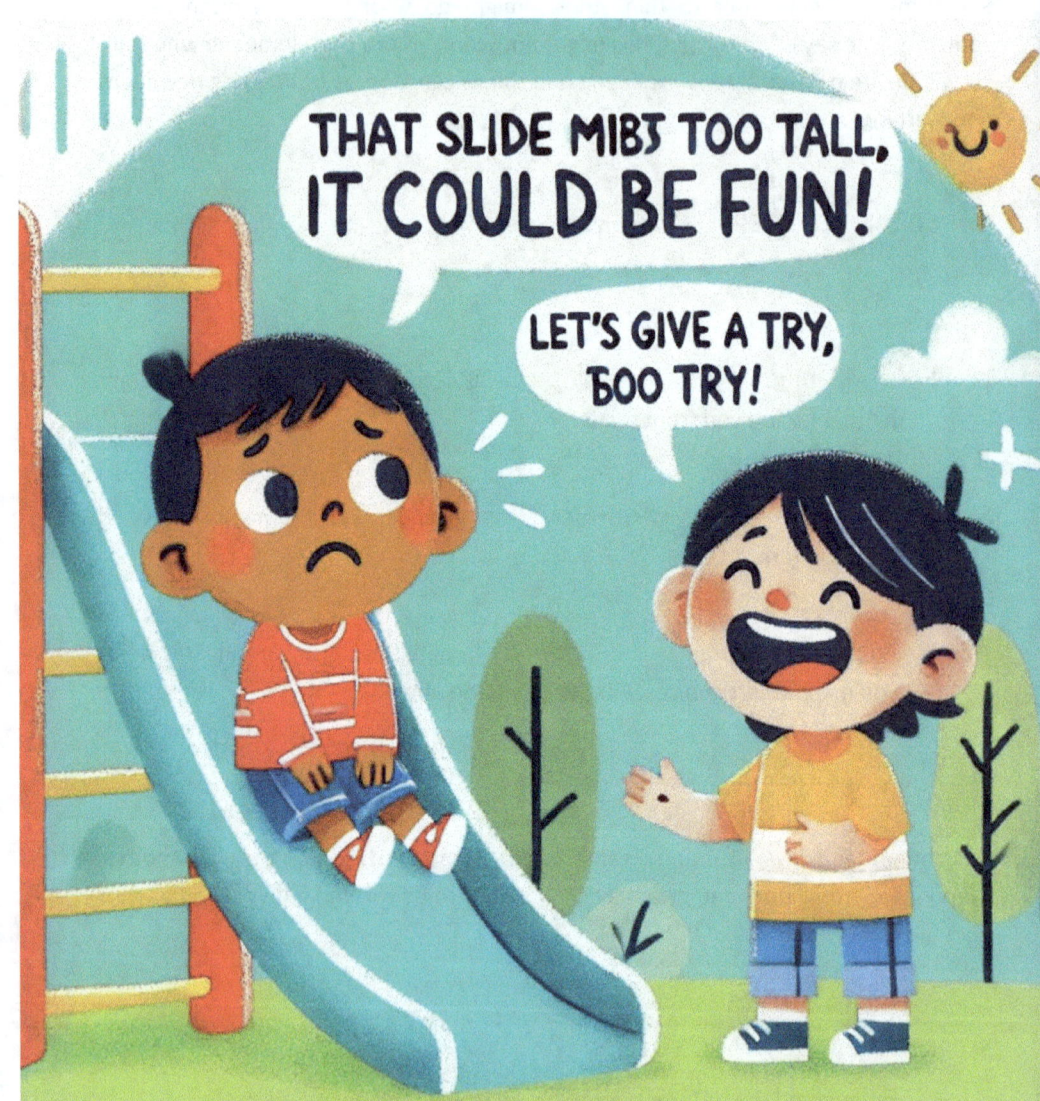

CHAPTER 18

WHEN YOU'LL BELIEVE ANYTHING

Sometimes, we believe things just because they sound nice, even if they're not true. Stories can make us feel a certain way and stick in our minds better than just numbers or facts. But it's important to look closely and ask, "Is this really true?"

THREE SIMPLE STEPS TO FOLLOW

❖ *Think About the Story:* When you hear something exciting or scary, ask yourself if it makes sense.

❖ *Look for Proof:* Find out if there's real evidence or facts behind the story, not just words.

❖ *Ask Questions:* Don't be afraid to ask, "How do you know?" or "Is there more to this?"

EXAMPLE:

Imagine hearing a story about a lucky charm that makes you win every game. It sounds fun, but is there proof? Winning takes practice, not just luck!

LESSON BREAKDOWN TO FOLLOW

- Stories are powerful, but they aren't always true.
- Always look for facts to see if a story is real.
- Ask questions to understand what's true.

The picture shows a child holding a "lucky charm" with great excitement while their friend says, "Winning takes practice, not just luck!" This shows that stories may sound good, but we should demand proof.

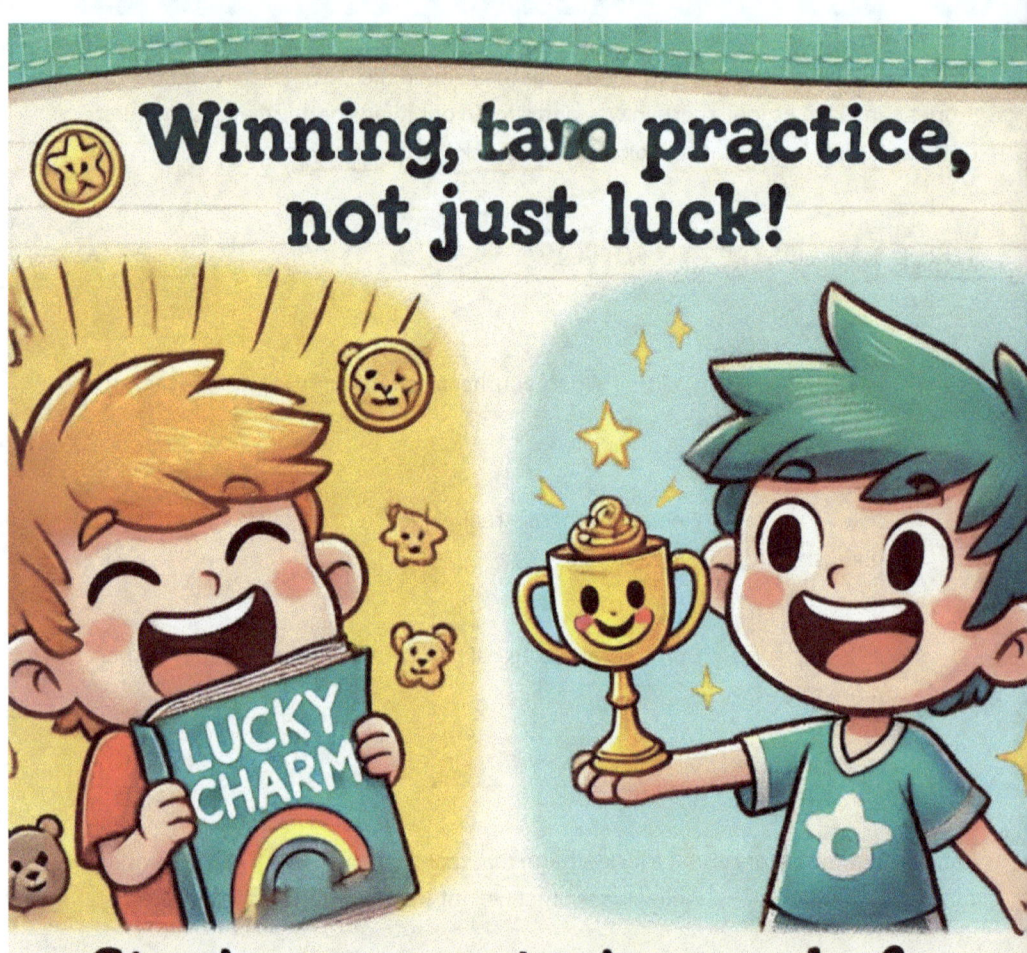

CHAPTER 19
ALL TOGETHER NOW

When it comes to how we handle our money, everyone thinks a little differently. The way we save, spend, or share money depends on how we've grown up, what we believe, and what we've learned over time. Understanding these things can help us make smart choices with our money!

THREE SIMPLE STEPS TO FOLLOW

❖ *Think About Your Choices:* Notice how you spend or save. Do you like to save up or spend right away?

❖ *Learn from Others:* Ask friends and family how they handle their money. You might learn new ideas!

❖ *Make Your Own Plan:* Use what you've learned to make a plan that works for you.

EXAMPLE

Imagine you get some birthday money. You could spend it on candy right away, or save it up for something bigger, like a game. Which choice matches what you've learned?

LESSON BREAKDOWN TO FOLLOW

- Money choices are personal; everyone handles it differently.
- Learning from others can give us good ideas.
- Making a plan helps us use our money wisely.

This picture shows two kids who handle money in different ways. One is saving it in a piggy bank and is having a great time buying small treats. This picture shows the lesson that everyone handles money in their own unique way.

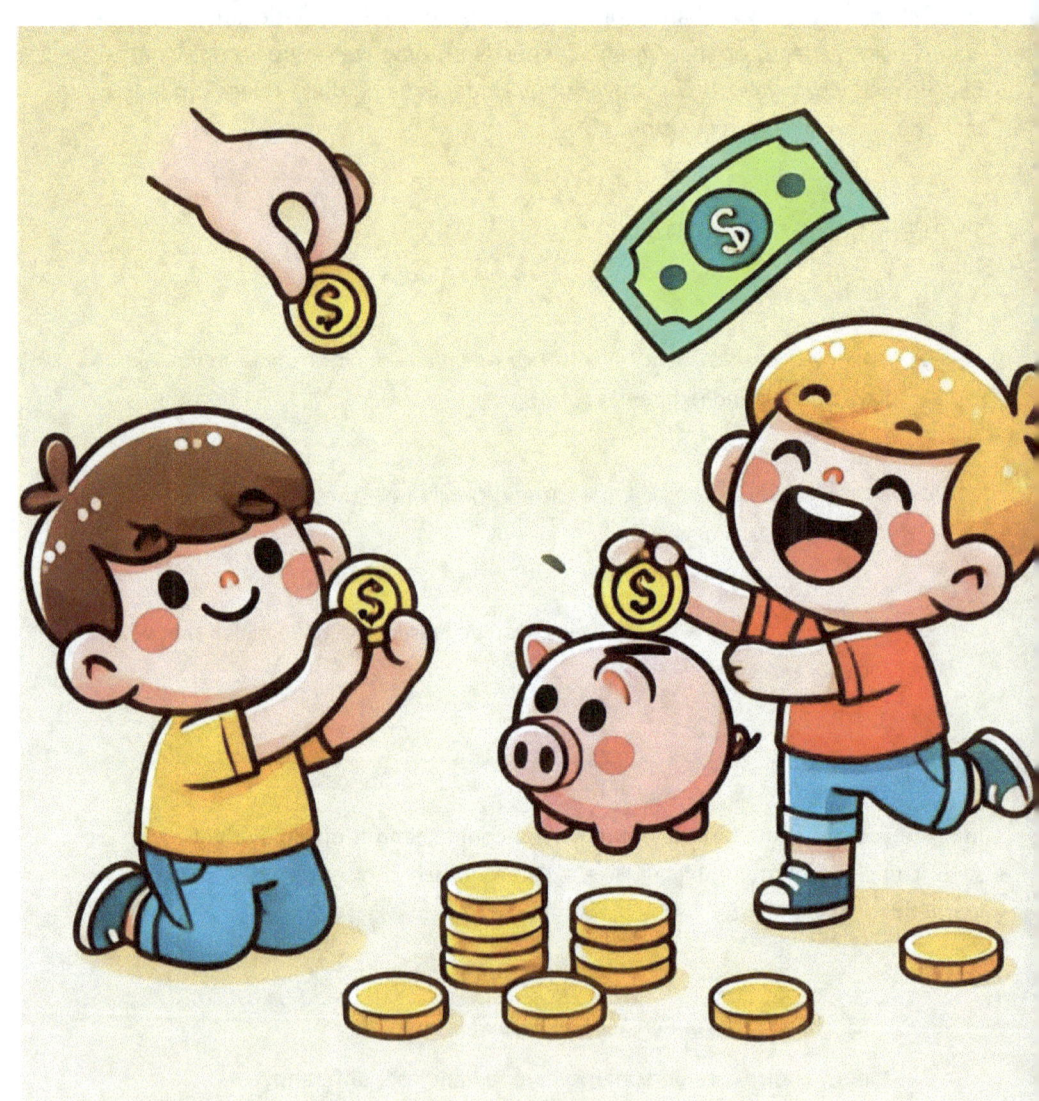

CHAPTER 20

MY MONEY THOUGHTS

"Understanding My Own Money Choices"

We all have our own way of thinking about and using money, and that's okay! The author's reflections help show that everyone's approach to money can be different.

LESSON BREAKDOWN TO FOLLOW

❖ *Recognize Your Choices:* Understand that everyone has their unique way of handling money. How you choose to save or spend money depends on what's important to you.

❖ *Learn from Your Choices:* Reflect on why you make certain money choices. Understanding this can help you make better decisions in the future.

❖ *Respect Other People's Choices:* Everyone's "money story" is personal. What works for one person may be different for another, and that's perfectly fine.

This lesson helps kids think about their money habits and understand that everyone's money choices are unique!

The picture for Chapter 20: Confessions shows a child holding a piggy bank with thought while another child spends a few coins on a snack. This picture shows the idea of making choices about your own money in a way that is clear and easy to understand.

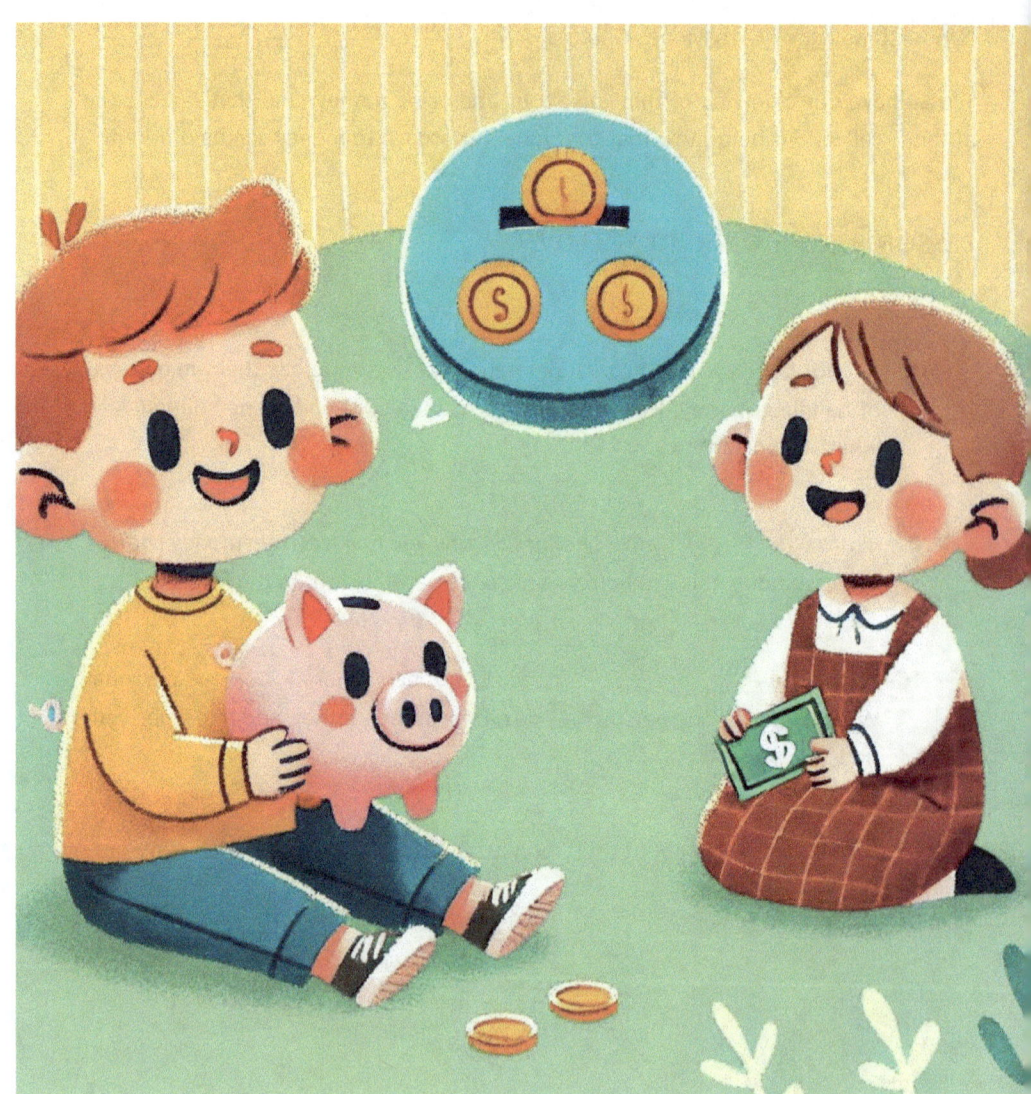

Best Recommendation

I highly recommend these three practical books on herbal remedies, complete with pictures and illustrations below. They make *wonderful gifts for family, friends, colleagues, and even doctors,* offering valuable insights for addressing various ailments naturally.

- Encyclopedia of Herbal Medicine Tea: Unlocking the Untold Secrets of Healing Plants for Every Ailment. *by Stephen B. Benson*

- The Holistic Guide to Wellness: Uncovering Secrets Big Pharma Prefers to Keep Hidden - Natural Herbal Solutions for Everyday Ailments *by Benson Stephen*

- The Lost Book of Herbal Remedies: Unlocking the Healing Power of Plants *by Wilson Benson*

Find them on Amazon or other online bookstores and discover the power of natural remedies!

www.ingramcontent.com/pod-product-compliance
Lightning Source LLC
Chambersburg PA
CBHW070340290526
45791CB00003B/1416